Surviving to Thriving

Surviving to Thriving

PAVING A NATURAL PATH
TO WELLNESS

KATHERINE A. BUTLER

ISBN: 1985850745
ISBN-13: 978-1985850743

DEDICATION

Benjamin Wang, M.D.
Thank you for trusting me to embark on this journey
and for monitoring my progress through it all.

FOREWARD

THE PROVIDENCE OF GOD!

Many years ago I met a beautiful, energetic little redhead that I immediately was drawn to. Little did either one of us know how much of an impact we would have on each other's lives.

Katherine allowed me to share my testimony of faith with her when she was having a particularly tough time, the first of several tough times she has been blessed to overcome. This was truly the beginning of a never ending friendship.

This book is a journey of experience, commitment, and the love Katherine has to help others.

Be blessed as you read this and share this with others who may need encouragement!

Myles Daniel

PREFACE

If there is one thing that I have learned, it is that we never get to where we are going in our own strength or on our own terms. There is always a team surrounding us; lifting us up, cheering us on, and some even making us stronger by trying to bring us down.

As more people began telling me to write this book, I struggled. The idea of using natural remedies; including herbs and essential oils, has come a long way in acceptance, yet still remains controversial. We appear to live in a world where people want to just take a pill for whatever ailment is bothering them. We want things fixed and we want things fixed immediately.

The more I thought about the idea for this book, the more I realized it is a major contributor to my testimony of faith. It is not about religion, rather a relationship. It is about trusting God and Him making provision in my life. It is Him guiding every step of this process and making provisions for my every need as they arise.

I am not a physician, I have never claimed to be, but what is found in the pages to follow is what has worked in my life. I am not saying nor will I claim the following to be a *'cure'*, but there can be potential to help others. What you will read in the pages to follow is about my personal journey. It is based on hours of my own research, trial and error, and making adjustments to reach the maximum potential for my own system.

Every day is a learning process and I am thankful for this. I did not want to create a highly scientific document, referencing a hundred different sources. I wanted this to be easily understood with simple instruction of what has been working for me and how it has made a difference.

I have had many people ask why I would venture out on my own and try to come up with my own treatments instead of trusting my team of diverse doctors and their specialties. Honestly, I began this journey of exploration because I was tired of the side effects from traditional Western medications. I was tired of being told that this was the treatment that I *had* to have, just to continue living. I wanted to move beyond surviving and finally be able to honestly say that I am thriving.

Katherine A. Butler

ACKNOWLEDGEMENTS

With special thanks:

- To my parents, for being by my side throughout every step, the ups and downs, and walking this journey with me. Thank you for keeping the comedy coming, trusting my decision to seek an alternate path, and for helping to lift me up when I fall (sometimes literally).

- To my brother, Joe. You help me to keep things in perspective. Thank you for being my sounding board and strength. I love you.

- To Dave, for loving me and volunteering to walk this journey with me. From sleepless nights to crazy moods and weird foods placed before you at dinner. Thank you for sticking with me through it all, when you have no idea what to expect.

- To Myles, for your love and friendship throughout the years. For knowing me before diagnosis and staying with me throughout every step and stumble of this journey. For sharing your testimony of faith and assisting in my exploration of alternative treatments. I am forever grateful.

- To Rachel and Donna, two friends encouraging this book and the documentation of my journey long before I ever wanted to start the project. If I had listened to you when you first encouraged me, this book would have been released months ago!

- To Kennedy, my herbal guide and life-long friend. Thank you for introducing me to herbs I had never even heard of or thought about. For being patient with me and teaching me how to use nature to help bring me from surviving to thriving.

- To all of my family and friends, thank you for never giving up on me when things got tough. For being there during the times I didn't even like myself or want anyone around. Thank you for the care packages, encouragement cards, calls, and visits. You kept me going and I appreciate you never giving up on me.

- To my readers, for following me through every publication and genre that has developed over the past eight years. This job would be pointless without you.
- To God, my Heavenly Father and the Great Physician, whom has guided me every step of this journey, caught me when I have stumbled, pulled me out of the darkest depths, as well as given me the hope and strength to keep moving. You are my Light and my Strength; I am nothing and I have nothing without You.

CONTENTS

1. WHERE IT ALL BEGAN

It has now been over eleven years since this journey began. The date was February 6, 2007. I had finished a shift at work, at a local gym, and my parents gave me no choice for going to the emergency room. In this moment, my life was forever changed and the dreams that I had for the future shattered before me.

I was feeling okay, just tired, but I attributed that to my work schedule. The only visible sign that anything was going on was swollen legs. They were like stovepipes by the end of the day. It started gradually; they would swell during the day and return to normal size overnight while I was sleeping. Little by little, the swelling didn't go down overnight. Each morning my legs were a little larger than the previous morning. Even living in Florida, I tried to hide my legs with long pants, say I was doing okay, and continue to carry on with normal activities.

This morning was different. I had no choice but to go and try to discover what was causing this. I couldn't go to my primary care doctor; honestly, I didn't have one at the time. I had moved to Florida five months prior and, the area where I was living at the time, just three months prior. Finding a doctor was not high on my priority list. I was twenty-eight years old and healthy. I didn't feel as though I needed to see a doctor.

Within moments of arriving at the emergency department, I was taken back to a private area and the testing began. In seemed like mere moments before we were told that my blood pressure was two hundred and thirty over one hundred and forty. I couldn't comprehend what was happening, I didn't even have a headache. I was diagnosed with Acute Renal Failure, Hypertension, Congestive Heart Failure, and a Bacterial Infection.

I recall lying there so frustrated. I was due back at work in just a few hours as I was working a split shift that day. Whatever these doctors were saying was obviously false and they must have switched my test results with another patient in the emergency department. I came in feeling well, just swollen legs. I was due back at work and I had my life to get on with.

I'm not certain what they gave me for medication, but I went to sleep. I was in the Intensive Care Unit (ICU) the next time I became consciously aware of my surroundings. Once I was awake, I received two units of blood due to low counts.

It was two days after my admission, once I was stabilized but still in the Intensive Care Unit, that I went downstairs at the hospital to have a kidney biopsy. It was determined that I had only twenty-eight percent function of my kidneys. Yes, that is out of one-hundred percent. They were failing, we didn't know how quickly, and at this point we still didn't have a known cause.

Every day I was wheeled around the hospital for multiple CT scans, x-rays, and ultrasounds. Each morning they did multiple blood tests and were usually back a few hours later to draw more because there were still no answers.

On February 12, six days after my admission, it came back that I had a positive Antinuclear Antibody (ANA) blood test result, which its purpose is to help diagnose autoimmune diseases. The next day it was confirmed that I had Systemic Lupus Erythematous (SLE).

I finally had a diagnosis, something I could work with. What the journey would entail was something I never expected.

2. THE JOURNEY

I was told that the first year would be the most difficult and the team of doctors were not lying when I was told this. The challenge would be finding the right combination of medications and dosages that would provide me with optimal health. Once we had a diagnosis before us, we sat down and traced symptoms back over a dozen years. Individual issues treated independently of each other and the pieces of the puzzle remained scattered.

Up until this point, I had sun sensitivity, causing major blistering before peeling. My hands and feet would swell and we attributed it to humidity. I had thinning hair, migraines, multiple ruptured ovarian cysts, hypoglycemia, fevers, popping and painful joints when I walked, hypothyroidism, and cycles of depression. I had been diagnosed with acute pancreatitis in my early twenties, which my doctors attributed to drinking because of my age. I tried to tell them that unless water and not alcohol caused it, they needed to look further. They didn't believe me and I was sent home. Just eleven months prior to diagnosis, I received a letter from Coral Blood Services in California. They told me that they were unable to use my most recent blood donation due to the presence of an unknown red cell antibody. When I called to inquire, I was told that there was a "clinically significant presence of an unknown antibody". All of these pieces were finally falling into place.

I spent a total of thirteen days in the hospital my first admission and was out for seven days before being readmitted and having to receive two more units of blood. Because of this transfusion and my blood pressure continuing to rise, I ended up in the Cardiac Intensive Care Unit (CICU). I was started on a continuous intravenous infusion for thirty-six hours, just to control my blood pressure. This admission lasted six days.

Four days later I ended up back in the emergency room. My legs were so swollen that fluid was literally "leaking" from them. I was diagnosed with third spacing, a condition that occurs when fluid in the body shifts from blood vessels to the area between cells, that normally does not contain fluid or only a minimal amount of it.

I was about three months into my diagnosis when headaches began intensifying in severity as well as frequency. There was a great disconnect between my thought process and the words coming out of my mouth. I knew what I wanted to say, but it wasn't coming out right. I was taken in for a MRI and it was revealed that I had a lesion on my frontal lobe. I was started on antibiotics and by the time of my second MRI, it showed not only the lesion on my frontal lobe; however, ten additional lesions on my cerebellum.

The medication I was receiving was changed and I was placed on fall precautions. My risk of falls was due to not only the brain infection but also the muscle weakness, and I was placed on complete bed rest. In turn, I acquired a blood clot in my left calf. I could not receive blood thinners because doctors were afraid I would bleed out in my brain. Physical therapy would not work with me because I had a blood clot, and still I remained on bed rest. I ended up having to have an inferior vena cava (IVC) filter placed to prevent the clot from moving into my heart or lungs.

I reached a point that I could not sit up or even roll over on my own. I couldn't stand and still didn't have the strength and flexibility to even give myself a sponge bath. I had a doctor literally walk out of my hospital room and tell my parents that I could go home to die because there was nothing more that could be done for me. Fortunately, I had another physician on my team that basically said we didn't need her and we were not out of options at this point.

This is what my life had become, going in and out of the hospital, visiting with more doctors than I could keep track of, and receiving treatments I had never even heard of. Tests and hospital admissions became so frequent that even the transport team knew me by name.

A year after diagnosis, I was facing my first of what would become five hip surgeries. Both hips have had total replacements, revisions, and the left side had an extra surgery to remove scar tissue build up that was pressing against nerves and causing drop-foot; a gait abnormality and difficultly lifting the front part of the foot due to weakness and nerve compression.

I was referred to a larger hospital with more specialists, two and a half hours away from where I was living. At first, things went well. I was seeing a Rheumatologist as well as a Nephrologist. When the treatment they prescribed wasn't working, the impact of this large hospital took its toll on my health. They were a research hospital. They wanted to keep me on medication that wasn't working and making me sick because it was 'research'. I decided I was not a lab rat and my health was more important than their research, so I fired the team at that hospital and was referred to a different one, this time four hours away from where I was living, by my local physician. Here, I have had great success and have met specialists that look out for my best interest and general well being.

Once I received the diagnosis of Systemic Lupus and became stabilized, there appeared to be a trickling down effect to the presentation of other autoimmune diseases. In 2010, I received multiple diagnoses including Fibromyalgia; Sjögren's Syndrome; and Raynaud's. Fibromyalgia is characterized by chronic, widespread pain, tenderness, and stiffness of muscles, joints, and even tendons. It is a disease and although there is pain and tenderness, it is not associated with inflammation. Fibromyalgia can be accompanied with issues of fatigue, sleep, and memory complications as well as mood disturbances. Sjögren's can best be described in one word: dryness. It is dryness of the mucous membranes, most commonly associated with the mouth and eyes. Raynaud's is a discoloration in the fingers and toes most commonly associated with cold temperature changes; however, it can also be triggered by emotional stress. The discoloration can include white, blue, and red, possibly leaving a sensation of numbness to prickly or stinging pain as blood returns to the extremity.

In 2015, I was diagnosed with Chronic Fatigue Syndrome. This was the most challenging to try and explain to other people. As soon as I would mention the name, most people tended to cut me off by saying, "Oh yeah, I get tired too." It is more than being tired. The level of fatigue is extreme, it is absolute exhaustion. It worsens with any physical or mental activity, but chronic fatigue doesn't improve with rest. It is unrestful, unrefreshing sleep that is also associated with loss of memory and concentration, headaches, enlarged lymph nodes, sore throat, muscle pain, and joint pain. Chronic Fatigue can be debilitating and isolating.

After multiple treatments for bronchitis, pneumonia, and pleurisy as well as extensive testing, a confirmed diagnosis of Bronchiectasis came mid-2017. I could barely pronounce it, let alone figure out what it was when I first heard the word. Bronchiectasis is a thickening of the airway walls as a result of chronic inflammation and or infection.

Around this same time, I also went through an extensive cardiac workup related to chest pain and shortness of breath with *any* exertion. I was admitted to the hospital, received a few doses of nitroglycerin, and was scheduled for a stress test. I honestly thought I was doing well; I went ten minutes on the treadmill. I wasn't breathing the best, but I still went ten minutes and felt it was an improvement from getting short of breath just walking to the mailbox at the end of our driveway. I am certain the doctor wasn't thrilled with me when I said it was ten minutes more than I normally do on a treadmill, but it was the truth. I was told they were going to finish my stress test in nuclear medicine; injecting a radioactive dye as well as a medication into my system that mimics exercise by increasing blood flow to my heart. Images were then taken to see if there were areas of the heart not receiving adequate blood flow. The result was that there appeared to be evidence of a previous myocardial infarction, a heart attack. Looking back, I am almost positive I know exactly when and where I was when this occurred; in 2006 while hiking Table Rock Loop Trail out to Grafton Notch State Park.

With all that was going on medically, I struggled to function. I was to the point that some days I was out of energy after just getting up in the morning, and there were days it took an hour to do even that. Something had to change.

I went to a local natural foods store and purchased some Lavender and Peppermint essential oils as well as a small diffuser. I was hoping that the Lavender would help me relax in the evenings and the Peppermint would hopefully help lift me up and give me a little energy. At the very least, I hoped that the combination would somehow help make me feel better during the day, although I wasn't exactly sure what that would entail.

It worked okay, certainly not a miracle, but the Lavender did appear to help me relax and sleep better and the Peppermint, if nothing else noticeable, helped keep me awake. During this time, I stumbled upon finding out that Peppermint essential oil was also beneficial in reducing nausea and upset stomach.

3. THE LAST ROUND

I will admit, my photo collage is deceiving; however, it plays in perfectly to the view from society upon those of us with autoimmune diseases as well as the cliché, "but you don't look sick." Even cruising around in a wheelchair, I didn't *look* sick. What I found interesting was that nobody asked why I was in a wheelchair. There were some looks of sympathy, judgment, rolling of eyes, and sighs, but still, nobody asked *why*.

This is my story, this is where I have been, the journey of more than a decade of my life. Overall, I have had a total of thirteen surgeries and thirteen rounds of chemotherapy within ten years of diagnosis. I have been unable to get around without a wheelchair three times and been dependent on using a walker six different times. At the time of diagnosis, I was spilling over five grams of protein in my urine within a twenty-four hour time period. To put this into perspective, there should not be more than one-hundred *milligrams* present. I have had more blood transfusions than I can even count and I was taking thirty-two pills per day when first diagnosed. Now, I only have four prescriptions, including one that is only once every four weeks, and can function throughout the day. It has been a long journey, but I have come to a point where I can honestly say it is one I would not change.

I am not sharing these things for sympathy; that is one thing I do not want. What I want is to share my experience in a way that you, as the reader, will be able to understand where I have come from and how far I have come. I want to provide others a glimmer of hope where there may seem to be none. I want others to understand this may be a possibility for their own health, one that they have not considered or even thought about. The following was my turning point.

* * * * * * * * * * * * * * *

I remember the evening. It was September 6, 2016 and I was spending the night at a hotel in Orlando. I had a dose of Rituxan earlier in the day, an infusion I had received multiple times before. This evening was different.

It was about nine in the evening and I noticed that my face and extremities were slightly swollen. I became chilled, I was slightly off balance, and there was some pressure in my chest. None of these symptoms alarmed me or were that far from common for me. It had been a long day, I was tired, and the sodium chloride solution with my infusion always caused some puffiness. I just needed to relax and I would be better in the morning. I didn't think much of the symptoms until I happened to look in the mirror and noticed the rash down my neck and across my face. I was having a reaction and had nothing with me to take in the hope of counteracting it. As I said, I had received this same medication multiple times before without issue.

Dave and his younger son, Adam, went down the road to the pharmacy to purchase some Benadryl for me.

While they were gone, I vividly remember sitting on the bed in the hotel room and breaking down to tears. I felt frustrated, defeated, completely broken, and came to the point that I talked to God like He was standing there in front of me.

"God, this isn't working. I am so tired. I can't keep doing this."
I paused. Waiting for a response, almost pleading for one, and got nothing.
Tears were flowing as I put my head in my hands and shook my head.
"God, what happens if this doesn't work? Where do I go from here? I'm running out of options."
I paused and within moments a feeling of calm washed over me. Two words stood out boldly in my mind.
"Trust Me."

"God, I do trust You, but..."
"Trust Me."
"Yes, but..."
Finally and very clearly it came.
"No buts. Trust Me. Period."
"Lord, I trust You and am counting on Your promises, I am trusting You to guide my very next step, whatever that may be."
With total surrender came a wave of peace.

In this moment, I realized that my emotions, my own hands, and my own strength could not handle what was happening to me…but my God could and would. As I thought this, a verse came to mind that I had known for quite a while but never consciously thought about so in depth as this moment:

"And we know that all things work together for good to those who love God, to those who are the called according to His purpose."
(Romans 8:28 New King James Version)

I grew up attending church, but I didn't believe in God because my parents told me to. I didn't believe in God because the church told me to, nor did either one force me to. I believed in God because I had already seen Him at work in my life. With what I had been through, I truly believe I would not be alive if it were not for His provision over my life. Bad things, sometimes even horrible things may happen, but He is with me every step of the way. Nothing comes into my life that He has not first allowed and that He will not be with me every step through. I have learned that trials are a testing of our faith; however, they are also there to prepare us for whatever we may face down the road of life. There is a reason for everything that happens, but we are never alone in our journey.

I don't know how much time had passed. The rash had spread down my chest by the time Dave and Adam returned to the hotel room. I had wiped the tears from my eyes, washed my face, and was sitting there like nothing had happened, but something had changed within me. I took 50mg of Benadryl. I didn't know what the next step was as I closed my eyes to sleep that night, but I was at peace.

4. A GLIMER OF HOPE

A few days later I was sitting around talking with some friends in the café at the church. One of them happened to mention that she was using essential oils and began explaining the benefits she was experiencing. It wasn't the first time the subject of essential oils had come up, but as I sat there, I began thinking about Frankincense and Myrrh, both in the Bible and with medicinal properties. I half tuned out of the conversation and thought back to my experience in the hotel. No questions, no hesitations, just trust Him.

It went against everything I had been taught, all of the schooling I had to receive my nursing degree and Bachelor of Science degree. I wanted to be a Pediatric Oncologist, I had spent years, prior to getting sick, learning all I could about Western medicine. I wanted to make a difference, a positive difference, in the lives of children. Now, all that I had studied wasn't even working for me.

I had to learn to trust Him, to trust what I couldn't explain, to not rely on science and studies to guide my steps. I had just enough light for the step I was on and that step was *complete trust*. I couldn't move forward without this.

5. A TEST OF FAITH

I knew if I was going to embark on a path of natural medicine, I had to be all in. I couldn't try it for a week, maybe a month, and keep switching back and forth. When I went home that afternoon from the café, I did a very general search on the health benefits of essential oils. The amount of articles and opinion sites I received was overwhelming. I thought about my own journey and one of the major organs affected by lupus has been my kidneys. I tried narrowing it down by essential oils beneficial to kidney function. Again, an overwhelming list appeared on the screen before me. If I was going to start, I had to start somewhere and this seemed to be as good a place as any. I tried to look for commonalities between what each article was saying. I started writing down names of specific oils mentioned that I could research individually later. The list kept growing.

During my reading the following morning, I came across a specific verse from Scripture. Although I had been reading the Bible for a while now, it was one that I was not aware existed and it shed a new light, a new perspective on everything I had been reading about and contemplating over with regards to embarking on the use of essential oils in my daily routine:

"Along the bank of the river, on this side and that, will grow all kinds of trees used for food; their leaves will not wither, and their fruit will not fall. They will bear fruit every month, because their water flows from the sanctuary. Their fruit will be good for food, and their leaves for medicine."

(Ezekiel 47:12)

As I sat there, my eyes kept focusing in on three specific words, *'leaves for medicine'*. There was a specific reason those three words were present and I was entering into this territory as a foreigner, naïve to the world that awaited me. If we could use leaves for medicine, for healing, than that was one more example of God's provision in our lives. If leaves occur naturally, why is a large amount of our medicines produced synthetically?

6. WHAT I WAS SEARCHING FOR

When searching for what brand of essential oils to purchase, there was a wide selection. In addition to basing it on my friend's testimony, of the benefits she was receiving from a specific brand, I also read about the processing of the oil; from how the plant was cultivated, if it was already diluted, and how it was bottled.

When it comes to cultivation, no matter if I was looking at plants grown in the wild or farmed, I wanted to try to make sure they were free from the spraying of pesticides. I didn't see a point in trying to receive the benefits of essential oils if the plants had already been sprayed with pesticides before harvest.

It may sound strange that essential oils would come already diluted, but it is possible. There are some oils that already come with added bases, fillers, or additives. In an effort to save money and extend the quantity of oil a company can bottle, they will mix the oil with less expensive seed, nut, or vegetable oils. There are companies that even go so far as to produce oils synthetically which, in my mind, defeats the whole purpose. In both cases, the bottles will still be full, just not up to the standard I would prefer for my own health or the health of those I love.

When it comes to packaging, all essential oils should be stored in glass bottles or containers. Because of the strong chemical compounds of the oils, they tend to break down and react with plastic. Also, it should not be clear glass. I wanted oils that were stored in cobalt blue or amber glass due to the ability of ultraviolet radiation to degrade the properties of the oils. When it came to labeling, I wanted to be sure that it listed the Latin name of the plant. It may sound a little obsessive, but I realized that simply saying, "Lemon Oil" or "Peppermint Oil" may or may not have any plant oil in it, the oil could simply be perfumed oil and not have the same therapeutic properties as "Lemon essential oil" or "Peppermint essential oil". Lastly, I wanted to be mindful of where the oils were stored. This matters because if oils are stored in high heat areas, even in the back of a box truck for shipping, heat will mess with the chemical composition, again breaking down the properties of an oil. Ideally, 1 would receive a little bottle of potent liquid that has been distilled from the flowers, leaves, or roots of the plant.

After about a week of further research, I went ahead and ordered a "starter kit" from an essential oil company as well as an Essential Oil Desk Reference. The starter kit I purchased came with eleven different essential oils. This provided me not only with a larger diffuser for my home but also the ability to start exploring other oils more in depth. The book proved helpful by being able to personalize my search by the specific type of oil or by the condition of interest.

7. LEARNING ESSENTIAL OILS

The following information is not going to be an exhaustive reference of the essential oils I use, rather a list of those I use most commonly. I will say that there have been times when I have an assembly of seventy-five different essential oils available to me in my personal collection. I certainly don't use this large of a variety on a regular basis; however, I enjoy the variety.

Cedarwood essential oil is one I use most frequently. The primary reason for this is that I have found it helps combat hair loss, which is common with Lupus. The running joke in our family is I can shed more than the dog, which is quite evident each time I vacuum the house or clean the shower drain. Another reason I like this essential oil is that I have found it to help drain the lymphatic system, keeping the lymphatic drainage flowing and reducing swollen lymph nodes.

Copaiba is an essential oil that I first began learning about after receiving my starter kit. I have not only found it beneficial as a pain reliever and anti-inflammatory, but also to help decrease anxiety levels.

Many people have heard of Eucalyptus and although this is a very general term, there are different types of Eucalyptus that I have found to have different benefits. For example, when I use Eucalyptus Globulus, I have found it to be most beneficial as a decongestant, for use with respiratory infections, as well as pain associated with joints and muscles. Eucalyptus Radiata on the other hand, although still good with respiratory issues, I have found it to be more beneficial as an anti-inflammatory verses specific pain. I have made blends combining both types with a carrier oil as they do have a different ratio and types of components.

The next three essential oils I am going to group together; Frankincense, Galbanum, and Myrrh. All three of these are referenced in the Bible. Myrrh is mentioned as early Genesis:

"And they sat down to eat a meal. Then they lifted their eyes and looked, and there was a company of Ishmaelites, coming from Gilead with their camels, bearing spices, balm, and myrrh, on their way to carry them down to Egypt."

(Genesis 37:25)

Frankincense and Galbanum are mentioned for the first time, together in the Book of Exodus:

"And the Lord said to Moses: "Take sweet spices, stacte and onycha and galbanum, and pure frankincense with these sweet spices; there shall be equal amounts of each."

(Exodus 30:34)

I use Frankincense and Myrrh primarily for their anti-inflammatory properties, while I use Galbanum for pain relief. I have actually made a lotion combining all three essential oils that has been beneficial when my back hurts or begins to spasm.

Lemon essential oil I have used most frequently to aid in digestion and to settle an upset stomach when I inadvertently consume gluten.

The benefits of Oregano essential oil, I have found to cover a wide variety of symptoms; from arthritis to aiding in the elimination of respiratory infections, as well as settling an upset stomach. I have found it to be very versatile and one that I always have available.

The last essential oil I am going to discuss here is Rosemary. Like Cedarwood, I have found this essential oil helpful in combating hair loss. In addition to that, I have experienced the benefits of it being an anti-inflammatory, helps regulate my blood pressure, and assists in mental clarity when my thoughts are quickly turning into mush.

These are the core essential oils that I use most frequently.

Other people may or may not experience the same benefits that I do and I am by no means saying that these are a cure. What I am saying is that they are working for me and my system right now in ways that are proving beneficial for my health and well-being.

8. HEALING FROM THE INSIDE OUT

Around the same time I began looking in-depth into essential oils, I was also referred to a digestive health specialist. After much testing, he recommended that I try a gluten free or Paleo diet. Although I trusted him as a doctor, I still questioned his opinion of gluten free. It appeared to be rising in popularity and I viewed it more as a passing fad or the going trend of the moment. Still, I had reached a point I absolutely could not eat without becoming sick and I was willing to try almost anything.

Gluten is more than just wheat, it is a general term for a protein that is found in wheat, rye, and barley. It is commonly found in such things as breads, baked goods, soups, pasta, cereals, sauces, salad dressings, malt, food colorings, and even oats can be contaminated because they are grown beside wheat, rye, or barely in fields. The entire concept of what I was eating was going to be changing.

I had one month until my next appointment and those four weeks were a self-experiment. I began with shopping for anything I could find that was packaged and labeled as gluten free. I stocked up on fresh fruits and vegetables and tried to carve a path of understanding for what I could and could not consume. I quickly realized food was never going to taste the same and I was already convinced gluten made it taste better. It may not have agreed with me, that was still yet to be determined, but it certainly tasted better. Most of what I first discovered was expensive, tasteless or even worse, and lacking in variety.

As much as I enjoyed cooking and baking, I lost that for a while when I began gluten free eating because I had no idea how to go about it. I soon spent a couple hours sitting at a local bookstore and going through gluten free and Paleo cookbooks. I quickly learned that although it exists, all purpose flour doesn't really apply to all purposes in the realm of gluten free cooking. My pantry is now stocked with eight other types of gluten free flour on a regular basis, sitting right next to the "all purpose".

I realized that if I was going to be successful in this adventure, I needed to learn how to adapt recipes in a hope of conforming to this new lifestyle. I quickly learned there is more to it than just exchanging the flour. Yes, that is one of those lessons I learned quickly through trial and epic failure. Gluten free is a completely different consistency, baking time, and taste. I purchased new cookware, bakeware, and utensils. Everything was beginning new and I wanted nothing that had already been contaminated in the kitchen.

To me, the proof was in how I was feeling. I reached a point that I could eat without becoming ill. Once I eliminated gluten, I realized the effect dairy and sugar were having on me as well. Throughout this experimental time, I limited my dairy intake and switched from regular white sugar to Truvia, a sugar substitute. I understand that this is not stevia, but I found that Truvia does not fluctuate blood sugar levels, which was important.

I was in Jacksonville for appointments and staying at a hotel. I had been on gluten free for quite a few months by this point. I had almost completely eliminated soda from my life. I didn't drink it often, but it still tasted refreshing on occasion. This particular evening in the hotel soda sounded refreshing. As much as I had heard in the news about aspartame, I still preferred diet soda over regular. I had a twenty-ounce bottle of diet soda that evening and had barely drank a third of the bottle when my hands began to severely tremor. It was also the beginning of an intense headache. For me, this could have been caused by a variety of reasons, but within two sips and the symptom worsening, I knew it was the soda. It was to the point I could not even hold the bottle and bring it up to my mouth smoothly.

Fortunately, I had Helichrysum essential oil with me, already diluted with sweet almond oil, in a roller bottle. One of the many benefits of Helichrysum is that it is an anti-spasmodic and has continuously worked wonders on my hand tremors. I had a Headache Blend with me as well, that was also in a roller bottle and contained Eucalyptus Radiata, Frankincense, and Peppermint essential oils with sweet almond oil as the carrier. The Helichrysum I rolled directly on my hands while the Headache Blend on my temples, across my forehead, and at the back of my neck. Within ten minutes my hands were back to normal and the remainder of the soda had been discarded.

At this point, I consciously try to eat Paleo, but always gluten free at the very least. A Paleo approach consists of the consumption of meat, fish, vegetables, and fruit. What it excludes is dairy, grains, and processed foods. I have also completely eliminated sugar and dairy from my diet. It is a style of cooking I never thought I would embark on; however, food is supposed to nourish our bodies, not make us sick. To me, the journey of this transition has been well worth it.

9. THE HERBAL CONNECTION

When I thought specifically about my kidneys, one indicator of their function is the amount of fluid I retain. I spoke about what I had been trying and thinking about with a close friend and he immediately sent me an article regarding dandelion as a natural diuretic. This was the beginning of my herbal journey in addition to essential oils and a healthy lifestyle.

The more I learned about herbs and their medicinal qualities, the more I focused in on my kidneys. The fluid retention, the level of protein in my urine, as well as their overall health and function were all concerns. The more research I did, the more I became interested in Dandelion Leaf, Dandelion Root, Stinging Nettle, and Yarrow.

Dandelion Leaf I use primarily as a diuretic, while Dandelion Root has been shown to assist in decreasing the amount of protein I spill. Stinging Nettle is one of my favorite herbs as I have found to be a diuretic, a detoxifying agent reducing the amount of protein in my urine, as well as an anti-inflammatory. Yarrow has more of a bitter taste to me, yet I continue taking it because I have found it to be beneficial in lowering my blood pressure, as an anti-inflammatory, and a mild diuretic for my system. A great deal of the benefits for essential oils and herbs that I use overlap, as I wanted a variety of options and not constantly having to take the same thing, especially when it comes to drinking tea.

Another issue that I was having was almost continuous

urinary tract infections. Every time I went to the doctors, I had another one and was once again placed on antibiotic. I soon focused my research on this specific problem and found Goldenseal. From what I was reading, it was said to be an anti-bacterial and help prevent this specific type of infection. It took some adjustments of the dosage, but I have found that a 570mg capsule twice a day has completely eliminated the infections from my system.

As I mentioned earlier, 2017 was a rough year for recurring Bronchitis, Pneumonia, and Pleurisy. It was like a continuous lung infection or collection of fluid. This was also when I was diagnosed with Bronchiectasis. To try and counteract recurring infections, I now take Red Clover as needed, in the form of hot tea. I have found this herb to be an expectorant as well as to help purify my body and rid it of lung infections at the slightest hint of one.

It was not that long ago that it was thought I had lymphedema, swelling in the arm or leg caused by lymphatic system blockage. My first line of defense was no longer what medication can I take to fix that, it was what oil can I use or what herb may help me get my lymphatic system back on track? That is when I added Cleavers to my routine. Cleavers, also known as Goose Grass, is common throughout North America and Europe, mainly found along roadsides. In addition to being a diuretic, it is also a great herb to help detoxify the body and drain the lymphatic system.

I am thankful for these herbs and others, for God allowing an understanding in my life of how they can benefit me specifically. I can't say that they will help everyone or even that they will have the same benefits for each person. We are all different, but this is what and how they have benefited my well-being.

10. WHERE I AM NOW

As I close with this final chapter, I do not want the reader to think that everything is perfect in my life. I still have ups and downs, I still have tough days, but I also have a lot more good days than what I have had throughout the past eleven and a half years.

At the time that I release this book, it has been twenty-one months since my last round of chemotherapy. I have learned more than I ever thought I would about essential oils and medicinal herbs. I have stepped away from all that I had studied in the world of Western medicine to discover something that would work for me. What I found was God's answer to my needs. I found nature, I found His provision, I found just enough light to take the next step forward only to find a door of possibilities open before me.

Since beginning the journey of essential oils and medicinal herbs, the medications I take have significantly changed. Aside from coming off quite a few prescriptions completely, the remaining few have each had their dosages lowered. Not only has the medication itself changed to be less taxing on my kidneys, the diuretic I currently take, Torseminde, has had its dosage decreased by half. Lisinopril is commonly used to lower blood pressure; however, I take because it helps to decrease the amount of protein I spill in my urine. That medication has also had the dosage cut in half.

I believe the most eye-opening change has been to my thyroid medication, Levothyroxine. It was twenty-two years ago I was diagnosed with underactive thyroid. Over the years, my dosage has been adjusted as necessary, always increasing. My most recent visit with my primary care physician revealed test results that I was taking too much medication for my thyroid. Up until six weeks ago, my thyroid medication has not decreased in twenty-two years. This result puzzled and excited me at the same time. Upon discussion with my physician, we found that I am eating healthier than what I was and also combining the use of Cedarwood, Frankincense, and Myrrh essential oils into my daily routine through homemade products. All of these factors assist in balancing hormones, including the thyroid. We will continue to monitor my thyroid levels to determine the proper dosage of medication and adjust as necessary.

I can honestly say that I have reached a point, knowing in my heart that if this journey was what I had to go through to become the person I am today, I wouldn't change it. I am even thankful for it. Let me make clear that I wouldn't have chosen it, I didn't choose it, but I wouldn't change it. I have learned it is our trials, our hardships, our pain, and more importantly our attitudes toward approaching them that helps to shape us. We need to try, we need to show up, and we need to keep moving forward each day. I didn't look in the mirror because I didn't like what I looked like, but I kept going.

It wasn't in spite of my faith that I was able to do this, it was because of it. I know that I serve a God who not only sent His Son to the cross for our sins, but He also meets us where we are. It is not a dozen different paths up the side of a mountain and we all end up at the same destination. He is the One who reaches down to help us up in the midst of trials, He goes to battle for us when we are too weak to stand on our own, and He surrounds us with the people we need in the moment to help get us where we need to be. I serve a God that is bigger than my diagnosis; no matter how many I receive. He has orchestrated my every breath.

We need to keep going no matter what the circumstances are and continuously choose joy. When I started this endeavor, I didn't know if this was going to work for me, but I knew what I had been doing wasn't working. I reached a crossroad and instead of giving up, I knew that the glimmer of hope along this path, what little I could see, was something worth trying. I do not focus on how difficult the journey has been, rather how much more difficult it could have been and would have been without Him. It is God who has made provisions in my life, in my every need, and for every step of this journey. I trust in that and it is how I transitioned from surviving to thriving.

"Help me, O Lord my God! Oh, save me according to Your mercy, That they may know that this is Your hand – That You, Lord, have done it!
Psalm 109:26, 27

Before entering this next section, I want to reiterate that the following information is what has worked in my life, with my specific system. Not everybody is the same and not everybody will experience the same results at the same level of intake. The following information is not intended to diagnose, treat, cure, or prevent any disease. What I do know is that the lifestyle changes that I have made as well as my faith in His hand over my life are what have brought me so far.

Trust in the Lord with all your heart, And lean not on your own understanding; In all your ways acknowledge Him, And He shall direct your paths.

Proverbs 3:5,6

MY SCHEDULE

ACTUAL PRESCRIPTION MEDICATIONS:
GAMMAGARD
- for Immunodeficiency
- 30,000mg Intravenously every four weeks

LEVOTHYROXINE
- for Hypothyroidism
- 88mcg tablet each morning

LISINOPRIL
- for Proteinuria
- 5mg tablet each morning

TORSEMIDE
- for Fluid Retention
- 5mg tablet each morning

OVER THE COUNTER AND HERBAL USE:
CALCIUM
- 600mg tablet three times per day

CLEAVERS HERB
- One cup of hot tea each week

DANDILION HERB
- I most commonly use Dandelion Root; however, I have also used Dandelion Leaves and Flowers.
- One cup of tea each afternoon

DANDELION ROOT
- Two 500mg capsules each afternoon

GOLDENSEAL ROOT
- 570mg capsule twice per day

MAGNESIUM
- 500mg per day

MULTI-VITAMIN
- One tablet each morning

SKULLCAP
- 850mg tablet at bedtime

STINGING NETTLE HERB
- One cup of hot tea each morning

SYSTANE ULTRA EYE DROPS
- As needed for dryness

TURMERIC
- 500mg tablet each morning

VITAMIN D$_3$
- 800 I.U. tablet three times per day

ESSENTIAL OIL USE:
- The type of oils that I use daily vary, depending on how I am feeling and what area I am most trying to focus on. Please see the Essential Oil Reference to view the most common oils I use.

MY MEDICAL HISTORY

❖ What I was diagnosed with and when

1996
- Hypothyroidism

2003
- Pancreatitis x 3

2007
- Systemic Lupus
- Congestive Heart Failure
- Acute Renal Failure
- Lupus Cerebritis
- Left Calf DVT
- Pancreatitis x 2

2008
- Avascular Necrosis (Bilateral of Hip Joints)

2010
- Fibromyalgia
- Sjögren's Syndrome
- Raynaud's Syndrome
- Pancreatitis

2013
- Pneumonia

2014
- Pleurisy

2015
- Pleurisy
- Gluten Intolerance
- Dairy Sensitivity
- Chronic Fatigue Syndrome

2016
- Bronchitis x 2

2017
- Pneumonia x 3
- Pancreatitis
- Previous Myocardial Infarction
- Bronchiectasis
- Immunoglobulin Deficiency

2018
- Lymphedema

MY SURGICAL HISTORY

February 8, 2007
- Kidney Biopsy

June 8, 2007
- Port-A-Cath Placement

June 26, 2007
- IVC Filter

March 11, 2008
- Right Total Hip Replacement

April 18, 2008
- Kidney Biopsy

September 16, 2008
- Left Total Hip Replacement

March 23, 2010
- Left Total Hip Revision Metal filings caused system to create an enzyme, in turn producing an acid. Acid deteriorated more bone. Replaced ball and socket (stem remains solid and in place), added a poly liner, ceramic head, two screws and bone graft to hold everything in place.

April 27, 2010
- Removal of Scar Tissue and filing off the tip of one screw that had shifted due to development of bone graft and both were pressing against the sciatic nerve.

April 22, 2011
- Partial Hysterectomy

December 5, 2011
* Kidney Biopsy

March 29, 2012
* Port-A-Cath Removed

June 7, 2012
* Right Hip Revision,.. Replaced ball and socket (stem remains solid and in place), added a poly liner, a ceramic head, three screws and bone graft to hold everything in place.

January 16, 2018
* Port-A-Cath Placement

ESSENTIAL OIL REFERENCE

❖ Below I will list the names of essential oils that I use most often and specifically what I most commonly use them for. Depending on the oil, I will dilute and run it in a diffuser, take in a capsule, or apply via roller bottles consisting of the essential oil and a carrier oil directly on the area of interest. Some oils are not meant to be ingested, so *please read the labels carefully*. Also, I use only pure essential oils and not synthetically manufactured or previously diluted oils.

BASIL
- Anti-bacterial
- Anti-Inflammatory
- Eases Migraines
- Use for throat and lung infections

CEDARWOOD
- Reduces hair loss
- Stimulates the Lymphatic System

COPAIBA
- Pain Relief
- Anti-Inflammatory
- Relieves Anxiety

EUCALYPTUS
- Expectorant
- Use for Respiratory and Sinus Infections
- Decongestant
- Soothes sore muscles

FRANKINCENSE
- Immune-Stimulant
- Reduces Inflammation
- Relives Respiratory Infections

GALBANUM
* Pain Relief
* Calms Nervous Tension

HELICHRYSUM
* Anti-Spasmodic
* Relieves Hypertension

LAVENDER
* Relaxant
* Relieves Muscle Tension

LEMON
* Immune Stimulant
* Aides in Digestion

LEMONGRASS
* Aides in Digestion
* Helps to Relieve Infections
* Promotes Lymphatic System Flow

MYRRH
* Anti-Inflammatory
* Anti-Bacterial
* Relieves Chapped and Cracked Skin

OREGANO
* Anti-Inflammatory
* Arthritis Relief

PEPPERMINT
* Relieves Headaches
* Aides in Digestion
* Reduces Nausea
* Relieves Arthritis Pain

ROSEMARY
- Anti-Bacterial
- Mental Clarity

WINTERGREEN
- Muscle and Nerve Pain

BLENDING OILS

FOR ARTHRITIS PAIN
- 10mL Roller Bottle
- 5 Drops Eucalyptus
- 10 Drops Lavender
- 3 Drops Peppermint
- 5 Drops Wintergreen
- Top off with Carrier Oil
- Gently massage into painful areas twice per day.

TO RELIEVE CONGESTION
- 2 Drops Eucalyptus
- 1 Drop Lemon
- 3 Drops Peppermint
- 2 Drops Tea Tree
- Diffuse or place in 10 mL Roller Bottle and top off with a Carrier Oil. (I have massaged it onto my chest and rolled it along the area of my sinuses and under my nose. Be careful not to get into your eyes.)

FOR HEADACHES
- 2 Drops Eucalyptus Radiata
- 8 Drops Frankincense
- 5 Drops Peppermint
- Diffuse or place in 10 mL Roller Bottle and top off with a Carrier Oil. (I have massaged it onto my temples, across the forehead, and the back of my neck. This is my go-to blend for all of my headaches, including migraines.)

TO BATTLE FATIGUE
- 4 Drops Grapefruit
- 3 Drops Peppermint
- 3 Drops Rosemary
- Diffuse

HERBAL REFERENCE

❖ The following herbs I have made into hot tea, iced tea, taken as capsules, and used in cooking. I have even added blue agave as a sweetener to a large batch of tea, cooled it, and made them into popsicles. The Dandelion Blossoms are the only herb that I have made into a jelly. Below each herb, I will list what I use them for and the benefits I have experienced.

CLEAVERS
- Diuretic
- Detoxifying
- Drainage of the Lymphatic System

DANDELION BLOSSOMS
- Great source of Antioxidants
- Vitamin A and B12
- Pain Reliever

DANDELION LEAF
- Diuretic

DANDELION ROOT
- Pre-biotic
- Detoxifying
- Decreases the amount of protein I spill in my urine.

GINGER
- Arthritis and Rheumatism Relief
- Relieves Nausea
- Relaxes Muscle Aches

GOLDENSEAL
- Anti-bacterial
- Preventative for urinary tract infections.

RED CLOVER
- Expectorant
- Purifying
- Helps rid my system of Bronchitis and Pneumonia.

SKULLCAP
- Insomnia
- Anti-spasmodic
- Support and nourishes the nervous system

STINGING NETTLE
- Diuretic
- Cleansing and Detoxifying
- Anti-Inflammatory
- Decreases the amount of protein I spill in my urine

TURMERIC
- Anti-Inflammatory
- Boosts Stress Tolerance
- Promotes Heart Health
- Supports Brain Health
- Supports Healthy Joints
- Soothes Digestion

VALARIAN ROOT
- Insomnia
- Anti-spasmodic

YARROW
- Lowers Blood Pressure
- Improves Circulation
- Reduces Fever
- Mild Diuretic and Detoxifying
- Anti-Inflammatory

RECIPES

BAR SOAP
- ❖ I use the melt and pour method when making bar soap, as I am not comfortable (at least at this point) working with lye.

- Soap Base
- Oils
- Herbs

- Cut off the amount of Soap you would like to use from the base.
- Place in a double boiler over low heat and melt completely.
- Remove from heat and add Herbs and Essential oils of choice.
- Pour soap into molds and allow to set 30 minutes in the refrigerator.
- Wrap individually.

BATH BOMBS
- 1 cup Baking Soda
- 1/2 cup Citric Acid
- 1/2 cup Epsom Salt
- 1 tsp. Water
- 2 tsp. Essential Oil
- 3 tsp. Olive Oil

- Place Baking Soda, Citric Acid, and Epsom Salt in a bowl and whisk together.
- In a separate bowl, mix together the Water, Essential Oil of your choice, and Olive Oil.
- Slowly add the liquid mixture to the dry mixture.
- Pack mixture tightly into bath bomb mold.
- Allow to dry completely.

BATH SALTS
- 3 cups Epsom Salt
- 2 cups Sea Salt
- 1 cup Baking Soda
- ~ ½ ounce Essential Oil

- In a large bowl, combine Epsom Salt and Sea Salt. Blend well.
- Add the Baking Soda to this mixture.
- Gradually add the Essential Oil of choice, making sure to not add too much as the salts will clump.
- Store in a dry, air-tight container.

BODY WASH

- ¼ cup Coconut Oil
- ¼ cup Raw Honey
- ½ cup Liquid Castile Soap
- 1 teaspoon Vitamin E
- 35 drops Essential Oil
- Glass Bottle

- Scoop coconut oil into a microwave safe bowl and heat on medium setting for 30 seconds until melted.
- Add Honey, Essential Oils of choice, and Vitamin E and whisk together.
- Add Castile Soap slowly, stirring gently to avoid creating suds.
- Transfer to Glass Bottle.
- Shake before each use.

DANDELION JELLY (It literally tastes like honey)

- 3 cups packed Dandelion Blossoms
- 4 cups Water
- 2 cups Sugar
- 1 box Pectin

- Using your thumb fingernail, cut and pluck the yellow blossom out of the tiny green leaves holding it. (Your thumb will get sticky and the flower will separate into petals.) Remove as much of the green as possible because green is bitter and turns the jelly green.
- In a medium saucepan, bring water to a boil. Add half the blossoms, stir. Cover. Turn off water and steep for 20 minutes. Using a fine mesh strainer, strain out and gently push on blossoms to remove some of the water. Add the same dandelion water back to saucepan and bring to a boil. Add remaining blossoms; cover. Steep 15 minutes. Strain out blossoms, pressing to remove water.
- Measure steeping liquid to 3 cups; add sugar, pectin, and bring to a boil, stirring until sugar dissolves. Boil for 1 minute, then skim off foam with a wooden spoon.
- Pour into hot sterilized half-pint jars leaving 1/4-inch headspace and process ten minutes in waterbath (in canner). Allow to cool completely while wrapped in a towels. Store in cupboard.

DISHWASHER DETERGENT

- ½ ounce Castile Soap
- 3¼ cups Purified Water
- 4 ounces White Vinegar
- 1 ounce Citric Acid Powder
- 1 cup Kosher Salt
- 20 drops Orange Essential Oil
- 20 drops Lemon Essential Oil

- Combine all ingredients until well blended.
- Store in Mason Jar.
- Use about 1½ - 2 Tbsp. of detergent per load.

ELIXIRS
- Herbs
- Honey
- Water
- Mason Jar
- Cheese Cloth
- Bottle

- Fill a mason jar about 1/3 full with Herbs of your choice.
- Pour boiling water over them, just enough to moisten the herbs.
- Fill remaining space in Mason Jar, up to the lip of the bottom of the rim with Honey.
- Allow to sit in a cool, dry place for about *four to six weeks*, shaking daily to mix.
- Strain through Cheese Cloth to separate the herbs from the liquid and pour into a bottle.
- Consume a teaspoon full once or twice per day, as needed.

HAIR CONDITIONER
- 1 cup Water
- 2 Tbsp. Apple Cider Vinegar
- 10 drops Essential Oil
- BPA Free Spray Bottle

- Combine all ingredients into spray bottle.
- Shake well before each use.
- Leave on hair 5 minutes before rinsing.

HAIR SHAMPOO

- 1½ cups Coconut Milk
- 1½ cups Liquid Castile Soap
- 40 drops Essential Oil
- BPA Free Bottle

- Mix all ingredients together in a bowl.
- Pour into bottle.
- Shake well before each use.

HAIR TREATMENT

- ❖ I use this between the shampoo and conditioner while others use it as a shampoo. It can be applied to wet or dry hair.

- 3 Tbsp. Baking Soda
- 9 Tbsp. Water
- 15 drops Essential Oil (Optional)
- BPA Free Bottle

- Combine all ingredients together and mix well.
- Pour into bottle.
- Shake well before each use.
- Leave on hair for 3 minutes.
- Rinse with warm water.

LAUNDRY DETERGENT TABLETS

- 4 ounce bar Castile Soap
- ¼ cup Baking Soda
- ½ cup Washing Soda
- ¼ cup Salt
- ¼-½ cup White Vinegar
- 5-10 drops Essential Oil

- Grate the bar of Castile Soap with the finest cheese grater you have available.
- Mix the grated Soap, Baking Soda, Washing Soap (see recipe), and Salt in a large bowl.
- Add the Vinegar a little at a time, mixing well after each addition, until it begins to clump and can easily be manipulated.
- Firmly press into ice cube size mold.
- Allow the molds to dry for at least 24 hours.
- Store in a Mason Jar.
- When you use, add tablet directly in with the clothes. They will not dissolve properly without enough water, such as in the detergent compartment.

LOTION

- ¼ cup Olive Oil
- ¼ cup Coconut Oil
- ¼ cup Beeswax
- ¼ cup Shea Butter
- 2 Tbsp. Vitamin E
- 40 drops Essential Oil
- BPA Free Lotion Dispenser Bottle

- Put Olive Oil, Coconut Oil, Beeswax, and Shea Butter in a glass bowl, then place that bowl in a saucepan with water.
- Heat burner to medium and mix ingredients together.
- Once mixed, put in refrigerator for an hour until solid.
- With a regular mixer or hand mixer, beat the mixture until it is whipped and fluffy.
- Add Essential Oils and Vitamin E.
- Mix thoroughly.
- Fill Container and store in a cool place.

SALT SCRUB
- 2 cups Coconut Oil
- 3½ - 4 cups Epsom Salt
- 8 – 10 drops Essential Oil
- Glass Jars

- Mix Coconut Oil, Epsom Salt, and Essential Oil of choice.
- Use amount of Epsom Salt to desired consistency.
- Spoon scrub into glass jars.
- Allow to cool before placing lids on.

SHOWER MELTS

- 2 cups Baking Soda
- 1 cup Citric Acid
- 2 Tbsp. Water
- 30-40 drops Essential Oil

- Mix together the Baking Soda and Citric Acid in a medium-sized bowl.
- In a small bowl, combine the Water and Essential Oil of your choice.
- Slowly, a few drops at a time, add the liquid mixture to the dry mixture and blend well.
- When thoroughly mixed, tightly pack into mold and allow to dry at least twelve hours before using.

SUGAR SCRUB

- ½ cup Coconut Oil
- 1½ - 2 cups Sugar
- 1 Tbsp. Essential Oil
- Glass Jars

- In a small saucepan, melt Coconut Oil over low heat.
- Slowly add 1½ cups Sugar and Essential Oil of choice.
- Sugar scrub texture should be dry enough to hold on fingertips. If mixture is too wet, add another ½ cup Sugar and mix.
- Spoon scrub into glass jars.
- Allow to cool before placing lids on.

SUNSCREEN (WATER-RESISTANT)

- ❖ This is approximately a SPF 20, for fair skin add an extra tablespoon or so of Zinc Oxide.

- ½ cup Coconut Oil
- ¼ cup Shea Butter
- 2 Tbsp. Non-Nano Zinc Oxide
- 1 Tbsp. Beeswax
- 10 drops Essential Oil (DO NOT USE CITRUS)

- Using a double boiler, melt Coconut Oil, Shea Butter, and Beeswax together until completely liquid.
- Stir in Zinc Oxide and Essential Oils
- Pour into small jar and store in a cool, dry spot.
- Lotion will thicken as it cools.

VAPOR RUB

- ¼ cup Olive Oil
- ½ cup Coconut Oil
- ¼ cup Grated Beeswax
- 20 drops Peppermint Essential Oil
- 20 Drops Eucalyptus Essential Oil
- Glass Jar

- Using a double boiler, place Olive Oil, Coconut Oil, and Beeswax.
- Heat on low until completely melted.
- Allow to cool slightly.
- Add Essential Oils.
- Pour into jars and allow to set.

WASHING SOAP

❖ Will assist in removing stains from clothing while washed.

- Preheat the oven to 400°.
- Make a thin, less than 1", even layer of baking soda in a pan.
- Bake the Baking Soda for 45-60 minutes, stirring halfway through.
- The texture of Washing Soap will be a grainier consistency and a little duller in overall color.

❖ For use when making laundry detergent tablets.

GLOSSARY OF TERMS

ANTIBODY
- A protein produced in the body to neutralize a toxin or other antigen.

ANTINUCLEAR ANTIBODY (ANA)
- Found in patients whose immune systems are predisposed to cause inflammation against their own tissue and body systems.

AUTOIMMUNE DISEASE
- A disease in which the body produces antibodies to attack its own tissues, including organ systems, leading to the deterioration and at times destruction of such tissue cells.

BRONCHIECTASIS
- Thickening of the airway walls as a result of chronic inflammation and or infection.

CARDIAC INTENSIVE CARE UNIT (CICU)
- A hospital unit specializing in the care of patients with various heart conditions that require continuous monitoring and treatment.

CHRONIC FATIGUE
- Extreme fatigue or tiredness that is not alleviated with rest and cannot be explained by an underlying medical condition.

CONGESTIVE HEART FAILURE
- A weakness of the heart that leads to the buildup of fluid in the lungs and surrounding body tissue.

DROP FOOT
- A gait abnormality and difficulty in lifting the forefoot due to weakness and nerve compression.

ESSENTIAL OILS
- A natural oil typically obtained by the distillation of the blossoms, leaves, or roots of a plant and having the characteristic fragrance of such.

FIBROMYALGIA
- A chronic disorder characterized by widespread musculoskeletal pain, fatigue, and tenderness.

GLUTEN FREE
- Food not containing a protein normally found in wheat, rye, and barley.

HYPERTENSION
- Abnormally high blood pressure.

HYPOGLYCEMIA
- A deficiency of glucose, a simple sugar, in the bloodstream.

HYPOTHYROIDISM
- Abnormally low activity of the thyroid gland.

INFERIOR VENA CAVA (IVC) FILTER
- A type of vascular filter implanted into the inferior vena cava, a large vein carrying deoxygenated blood to the hearts from the lower body, to prevent life-threatening pulmonary emboli.

INTENSIVE CARE UNIT (ICU)
- A hospital unit in which patients who are dangerously ill are kept under constant observation.

LESION
- A region of an organ or tissue that has suffered damage through injury or disease.

LYMPHATIC SYSTEM

- The network of vessels through which lymph, a colorless fluid containing white blood cells, drains from surrounding tissues into the blood.

LYMPHEDEMA

- Localized fluid retention and tissue swelling, most commonly in the arms or legs, usually caused by a blockage in the lymphatic system.

MEDICINAL HERBS

- Remedies and medicines made from plants.

NEPHROLOGIST

- A physician who studies and deals with the diagnosis and management of kidney disease.

PALEO DIET

- A diet based on the consumption of meat, fish, vegetables, and fruit, while excluding dairy, grains, and processed foods.

PANCREATITIS

- Inflammation of the pancreas.

PLEURISY

- Inflammation of the lining around the lungs, the pleura, causing pain when breathing.

PROTEINURIA

- The presence of abnormal quantities of protein in the urine, often indicating kidney damage.

RAYNAUD'S

- A condition resulting in the discoloration of fingers and/or toes when a person is exposed to temperature changes, most often cold.

RENAL FAILURE

- The loss of kidney function that can be either acute, occurring suddenly, or chronic, over an extended period of time.

RHEUMATOLOGIST

- A physician who specializes in the detection and treatment of musculoskeletal disease and systemic autoimmune conditions most commonly referred to as rheumatic diseases.

SJÖGREN'S SYNDROME

- A chronic inflammatory autoimmune disease characterized by dryness of the mucous membranes, especially of the eyes and mouth.

SYSTEMIC LUPUS ERYTHEMATOUS (SLE)

- An autoimmune disease in which the body's immune system mistakenly attacks healthy tissue, affecting any organ system.

THIRD SPACING

- A shifting of fluid in the body from the blood vessels to the area between cells, that normally does not contain fluid or only a minimal amount of it.

BOOKS

Ballantyne, Sarah. (2013). *The Paleo Approach: Reverse Autoimmune Disease and Heal Your Body.* Las Vegas, NV: Victory Belt Publishing Inc.

Ballantyne, Sarah. (2014). *The Paleo Approach Cookbook: A Detailed Guide to Heal Your Body and Nourish Your Soul.* Las Vegas, NV: Victory Belt Publishing Inc.

Chevallier, Andrew. (2016). *Encyclopedia of Herbal Medicine.* New York, NY: DK Publishing.

Johnson, R.L., Foster, S., Dog, T.L., & Kiefer, D. (2010). *Guide to Medicinal Herbs.* Washington, D.C.: National Geographic Partners.

Thomas, Donald E. (2014). *The Lupus Encyclopedia.* Baltimore, MD: Johns Hopkins University Press.

Life Science. (2014). *Essential Oils Desk Reference Sixth Edition.* Life Science Publishing.

Morse, Robert. (2004). *The Detox Miracle Sourcebook: Raw Foods and Herbs for Complete Cellular Regeneration.* Chino Valley, Arizona: Kalindi Press.

RESOURCES

BULK APOTHECARY
- 125 Lena Drive
  Aurora, OH 44202
- 888.728.7612
- www.bulkapothecary.com

dōTERRA
- 389 South 1300 West
  Pleasant Grove, UT 84062
- 800.411.8151
- service@doterra.com

EDENS GARDEN
- 1322 Calle Avanzado
  San Clemente, CA 92673
- 949.388.1999
- edensgarden.com

FRESH OFF THE FARM
- 495 Commercial Street
  Rockport, Maine
- 207.236.3260

MOUNTAIN ROSE HERBS
- P.O. Box 50220
  Eugene, OR 97405
- 800.879.3337
- www.mountainroseherbs.com

NATIVE SUN
- 11030 Baymeadows Road,
  Jacksonville, Florida 32256
- 904.260.2791
- www.nativesunjax.com

YOUNG LIVING

- Thanksgiving Point Business Park
  3125 Executive Parkway
  Lehi, UT 84043
- 800.371.3515
- youngliving.com

"And my God shall supply all your need according to His riches in glory by Christ Jesus. Now to our God and Father be glory forever and ever. Amen."
Philippians 4:19,20

PREVIOUS WORKS

Moving Forward (2010)

Stepping Stones: A Collection of Poetic Insight (2011)

Turing Point: A Book 'n' Blog (2011)

A Slice of Family History: Butler-DeRocle Cookbook (2012)

Letters from War (2013)

Pearls of Wisdom, Book One: The Pearls Series (2014)

Pearls of Hope, Book Two: The Pearls Series (2014)

Pearls of Strength, Book Three: The Pearls Series (2014)

Pearls of Commitment, Book Four: The Pearls Series (2015)

Pearls of Truth, Book Five: The Pearls Series (2016)

Pearls of Understanding, Book Six: The Pearls Series (2017)

Pearls I (2017)
- *Pearls of Wisdom, Pearls of Hope, and Pearls of Strength*

Pearls II (2017)
- *Pearls of Commitment, Pearls of Truth, and Pearls of Understanding*